THE POCKET GUIDE TO CPR FOR INFANTS AND CHILDREN

THE POCKET GUIDE TO CPR FOR INFANTS AND CHILDREN

GLORIA BLATTI, R.N., ED.D.

POCKET BOOKS
New York London Toronto Sydney Tokyo Singapore

An *Original* Publication of POCKET BOOKS

POCKET BOOKS, a division of Simon & Schuster Inc.
1230 Avenue of the Americas New York, NY 10020

ISBN: 0-671-00975-3

First Pocket Books printing April 1998

10 9 8 7 6 5 4 3 2 1

POCKET and colophon are registered trademarks of Simon & Schuster Inc.

Cover design by Brigid Pearson

Printed in the U.S.A.

Special thanks to:

Harriet Foreman, R.N., Ed.D. (Editing)

Daniel Crowley (Photography)
Dylan Crowley
Nicholas Blatti
Jacob Rek (Baby in photo)
Lisa Rek (Mother in photo)
Justin Blatti
Jillian Blatti

CONTENTS

3 CHOKING

4 QUICK REFERENCE

AUTHOR'S FOREWORD: THE ABC'S OF CPR

Over more than seventeen years of practice as a registered nurse (RN), I have attempted to resuscitate many children. Some have been "saves" and some, unfortunately, have died. It is impossible to describe the feelings of elation and humility following a save. To have a child or a parent look at you and thank you for being there at a time when they needed you most is a feeling second to none other.

Dr. C. Everett Koop, former Surgeon General of the United States, said, "If a disease were killing our children in the same proportions that accidents are, people would be outraged and demand that this killer be stopped!" Many of the accidents he referred to were choking on foreign objects and drownings that occurred in the absence of an adult adept in lifesaving techniques including and perhaps especially cardiopulmonary resuscitation (CPR).

As an RN and a mother, I am fully aware of the time constraints placed on parents, especially working parents, in today's hectic world. Nevertheless, I am a strong advocate of all parents taking the time to learn CPR. Your children's lives may depend on it.

The best way to learn CPR is to participate in a certified class. But as time goes by, skills will likely get rusty. This manual has been prepared to refresh your memory. In an emergency, this manual may also be used by those untrained in the skills of CPR.

—*Gloria Blatti*

HOW TO USE THIS MANUAL

This manual is designed to help you further understand the theory of infant and child CPR and to refresh your skills.* It also will aid you in understanding the sometimes mysterious workings of the human body insofar as breathing and heartbeat are concerned. And you will be able to learn some techniques to be employed in the event your infant or child chokes on a foreign object, and thus prevent the need to apply CPR.

A quick review of the Contents will assist you in determining how the manual is organized. An introduction is stated at the beginning of each

*Although CPR may be applied to people of all ages, unless otherwise stated, infants and children will be the reference points in this manual.

chapter and bold-faced type is used throughout to highlight areas of particular importance.

Pictures of CPR being performed on children are included to help you visualize crucial points. Reading the text and referring to the photographs will help fix the images in your mind in case you need to perform CPR. Remember to review the contents of the manual regularly and even conduct "dry runs" so that you can react with speed and skill if the moment for you to do so arises.

1

HOW DOES THE BODY WORK?

In order to effectively perform **CPR,** you need to know and understand the workings of the heart and lungs.

This chapter will explain how the heart pumps blood when you apply compressions (press on the infant's or child's chest) and how you give an infant or child air when you breathe into his or her mouth.

The Heart

If a child's heart stops beating, you will have to start pumping his heart for him. The diagram to the right shows you where the heart is located in the chest: under and to the left of the breastbone. The heart pumps blood to the lungs, where it picks up oxygen and then carries the oxygen to all parts of the body. Oxygen is needed by all body cells to carry out their functions. If the heart stops, oxygen will not be sent to the vital organs. After a very few minutes without oxygen, these organs will begin to die.

CPR is a technique used to keep the blood moving from the heart to the lungs (where it picks up oxygen) and then to the rest of the body. The most important

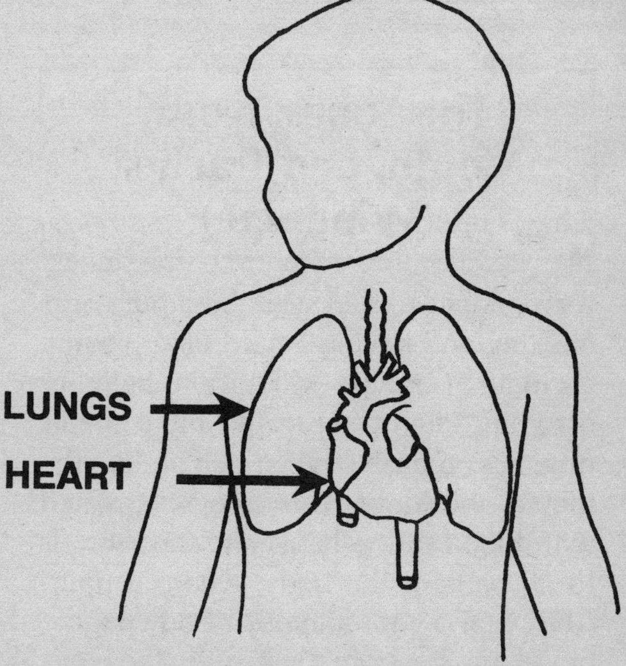
LUNGS
HEART

place it brings oxygen to is the brain, which *must* have oxygen within three to four minutes to survive.

The Lungs, Nose, Mouth, and Trachea (Windpipe)

If an infant or child stops breathing or is choking and having a hard time moving air in and out, you will have to help her breathe. When you breathe into a child's mouth, you push oxygen-rich air into the mouth and lungs. This oxygen is mixed with blood in the lungs and then travels to all parts of the body, where it nourishes vital organs and other body parts.

This diagram shows you where to place your hand on your child when performing **CPR.**

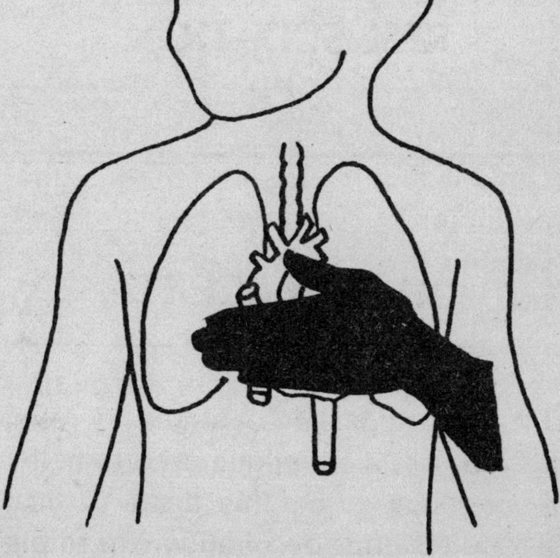

2

CARDIOPULMONARY RESUSCITATION CPR

What Is CPR?

CPR is short for **cardiopulmonary resuscitation.** It is a technique used to help a person breathe and his heart to beat, thereby restoring respiration (breathing) and circulation of vital blood in the body.

CPR is an action you can take to save a child's (or an adult's) life.

This chapter will help you to know when, whom, and how to call for help.

REMEMBER:

ACCIDENTS KILL!

One in three deaths among children results from injury!

In the United States, INJURIES are the number one cause of death in children from birth to fourteen years of age!

Children need us to make their environment to be as safe as possible. Unfortunately, children get hurt even when you are extremely careful. As a parent, life-threatening injuries will cause you fright, uncertainty, and an overwhelming need to respond. This manual is intended to help prepare you for the worst. Hopefully, you will never need to apply **CPR;** however, learning how to perform this skill can save your child's life.

Techniques for infant and child **CPR** differ slightly; therefore, the skills will be shown separately. Your understanding of this technique can help reduce the chances of your child dying from injury.

When to Use CPR

Cardiopulmonary resuscitation is a combination of mouth-to-mouth breathing and chest compressions that you can perform on your child until medical help arrives. It keeps oxygen-rich blood flowing to the child's vital organs (brain, lungs, kidneys, liver, etc.).

There are several reasons an infant or child may need **CPR:**

- Choking (if you are unable to dislodge the object)
- Drowning
- Allergic reactions that lead to cardiac arrest
- Suffocation
- Falling
- Electrical shock
- Children born with malformed airways
- Serious asthma
- Severe automobile accident
- Inhaling smoke or fire
- Poisoning

REMEMBER: ANY ONE OF THESE CONDITIONS OR SITUATIONS CAN HAPPEN TO YOUR CHILD. KNOWING *CPR* CAN MAKE A DIFFERENCE.

Whom Do I Call for Help? How?

Knowing how to call for help is just as important as knowing **CPR.** You will have to start **CPR** before help arrives, but be sure to call 9-1-1 for the Emergency Medical System.

Lifesaving Steps

1. If after one minute no one comes to your aid when you are trying to save your baby, then you must call for help yourself. Call 9-1-1.

2. It is very important to know the an-

swers to the following questions before a crisis arises:

How do I contact the emergency services?

What is the name and number of the child's physician?

What hospital does this physician routinely go to?

What is the Poison Control Center's number?

3. Decide where you will post the emergency numbers. Most parents find it easiest to keep them next to the phone. Keep your address and names of cross streets on this information card. Note your own telephone number on the card.

4. Tell the trained person on the phone what happened.

5. *Do not hang up!* You should be the last one to hang up the telephone.

CALL 9·1·1

REMEMBER: IN MOST COMMUNITIES, THE NUMBER TO CALL FOR HELP IS **9-1-1.** IF YOU ARE UNSURE, CHECK YOUR TELEPHONE BOOK OR CALL THE OPERATOR **NOW,** BEFORE AN EMERGENCY HAPPENS. KNOWING THE RIGHT NUMBER WILL GET YOU THE HELP YOU NEED QUICKLY TO SAVE YOUR BABY'S LIFE.

SAMPLE TELEPHONE CONVERSATION BETWEEN A PARENT AND 9-1-1

MOTHER: Help! My baby's choking!!

9-1-1: Please tell me what's happening.

MOTHER: I gave him a pretzel and he's choking!

9-1-1: Is the baby breathing?

MOTHER: Yes, but he's choking.

9-1-1: Don't try to get the pretzel out. Let him try to do it himself. What is your address?

MOTHER: Twenty-eighth Street and Park Avenue. One fifteen—the fifth floor. Please help me, I'm afraid . . .

9-1-1: What is your apartment number?

MOTHER: Nineteen.

9-1-1: Don't hang up. We're on our way. . . . How is the baby now?

MOTHER: My god, . . . he just threw up and he's breathing better.

9-1-1: That's great. We'll be there in just a few minutes.

Steps of CPR
AS EASY AS ABC

It is easiest to remember the steps of **CPR** by thinking of the ABCs. It is amazing how this simple memory tickler works.

REMEMBER:

A = AIRWAY

B = BREATHING

C = COMPRESS

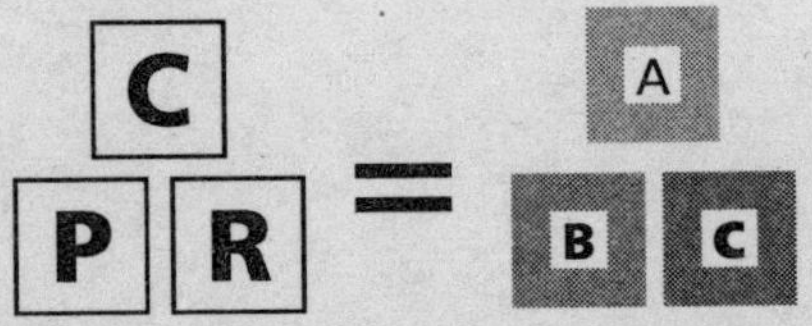

Infant CPR
UNDER ONE YEAR

CALL FOR HELP!
DIAL 9·1·1

STEP 1

FIND OUT IF THE BABY IS BREATHING

GENTLY SHAKE OR PINCH THE BABY

IF NO RESPONSE, PLACE BABY ON TABLE OR OTHER HARD SURFACE

STEP 2

A = AIRWAY

▶ *OPEN AIRWAY*

Place one hand on the baby's forehead and position two fingers of the other hand under the baby's chin. Gently tilt the baby's head back and pull the chin down. This pulls the baby's tongue off the back of the throat and opens the windpipe.

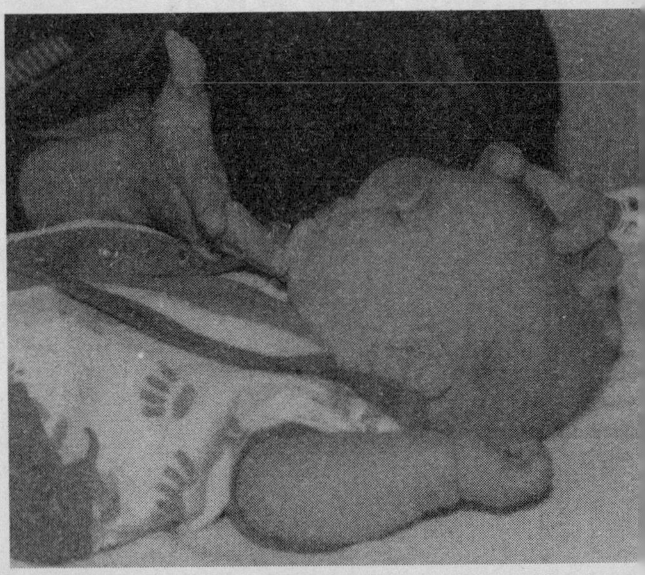

STEP 3

B = BREATHING

SEE IF THE BABY IS BREATHING

LOOK To see if the baby's chest is moving up and down.

LISTEN With the baby's head tilted back, put your ear near the baby's mouth and nose and listen for the sounds of breathing.

FEEL If there is air coming OUT of the baby's mouth onto your face, gently place your head on the baby's chest to feel it rise and fall.

STEP 4

IF THE BABY IS NOT BREATHING, BEGIN RESCUE BREATHING

While continuing to gently press on the baby's forehead with one hand and on the baby's chin with the other hand, cover the baby's mouth and nose with

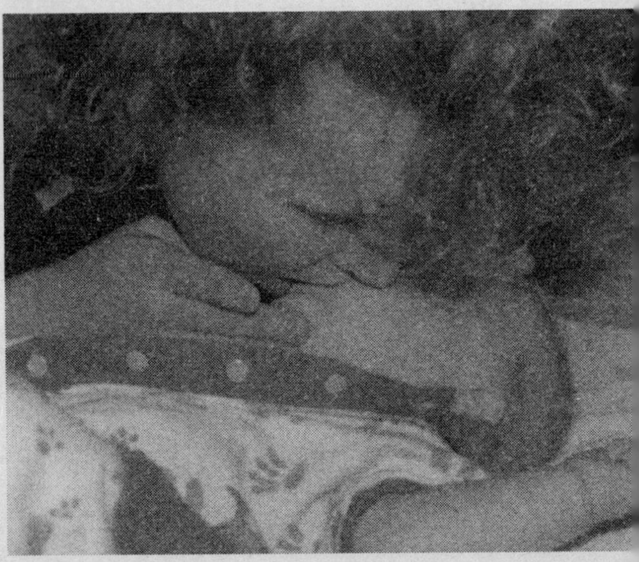

your mouth. Seal your lips firmly against the baby's skin to create a seal and prevent air from escaping.

Give two slow, strong breaths—enough to make the chest rise.

If the chest does not rise,

reopen the airway and follow steps 2, 3, and 4 one more time. Again, see if the baby is breathing.

C = COMPRESS

If the baby is not breathing, place your head on the infant's chest and listen for a heartbeat. If there is no heartbeat, start chest compressions.

STEP 5

NEVER START COMPRESSIONS IF THERE IS A HEARTBEAT!

▶ *CHEST COMPRESSIONS*

Remember to keep breathing for your baby in between doing chest compressions in order to move the baby's blood from the heart to the vital organs and the rest of the body.

With the baby on a firm surface, draw a make-believe line between the nipples.

Place your thumb and index finger just below the make-believe line on the baby's chest.

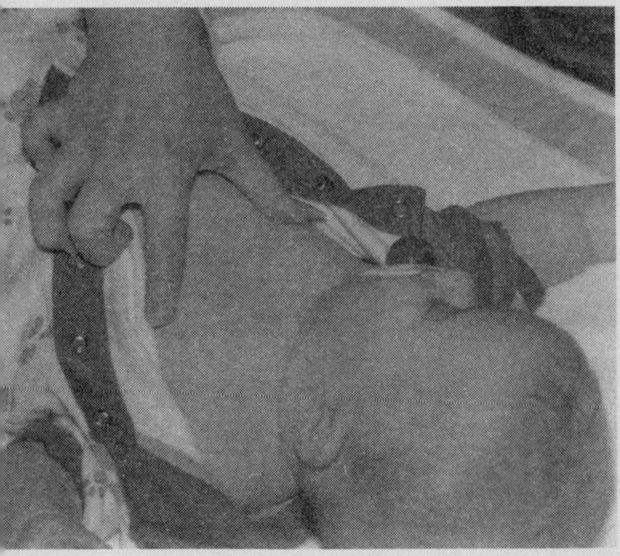

Push down on the chest about 1 inch.

Let the chest come back up.

Do this 5 times.

Then breathe for the baby as you did before: Cover the baby's nose and mouth with your mouth, being sure to make a tight seal, and breathe strongly enough to make the chest rise. (See **Step 4.**)

After 1 minute of doing this process, check to see if there is a heartbeat.

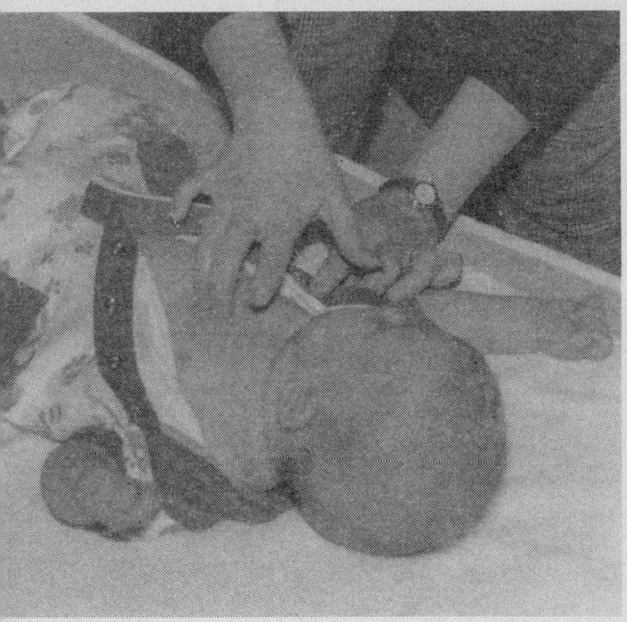

HELPFUL HINT

While Doing Compressions, Count Out Loud:

ONE • TWO • THREE • FOUR • FIVE • THEN BREATHE;

ONE • TWO • THREE • FOUR • FIVE • THEN BREATHE.

Child CPR
1–8 YEARS

THE STEPS OF CHILD CPR ARE SIMILAR TO THE STEPS OF INFANT CPR, WITH A FEW VARIATIONS. THE ABCs REMAIN THE SAME.

CALL FOR HELP!

DIAL 9 · 1 · 1

STEP 1

A = AIRWAY

TRY TO FIND OUT WHAT HAPPENED TO THE CHILD.

Shake the child. Ask: *"Are you okay?"* If the child doesn't answer, go to STEP 2.

STEP 2

OPEN THE CHILD'S AIRWAY

Lift the chin up, push down on the forehead, and tilt the head back.

B = BREATHING

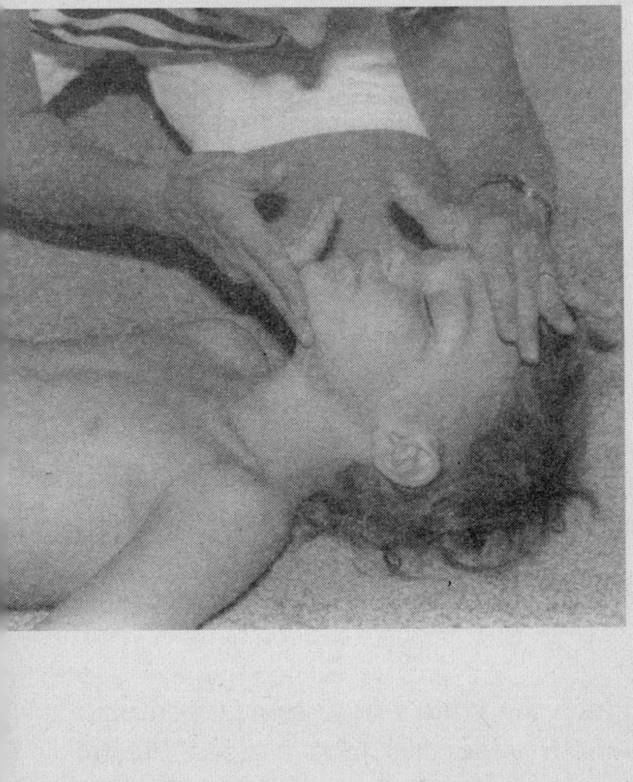

STEP 3

PLACE YOUR HEAD NEXT TO THE CHILD'S MOUTH.

LOOK at the child.

LISTEN to hear if the child is breathing.

FEEL if chest is moving. If the child is not breathing, proceed to STEP 4.

STEP 4

Pinch the child's nose shut. Open your mouth wide and take a deep breath. Breathe fully into the child's mouth. Give two breaths.

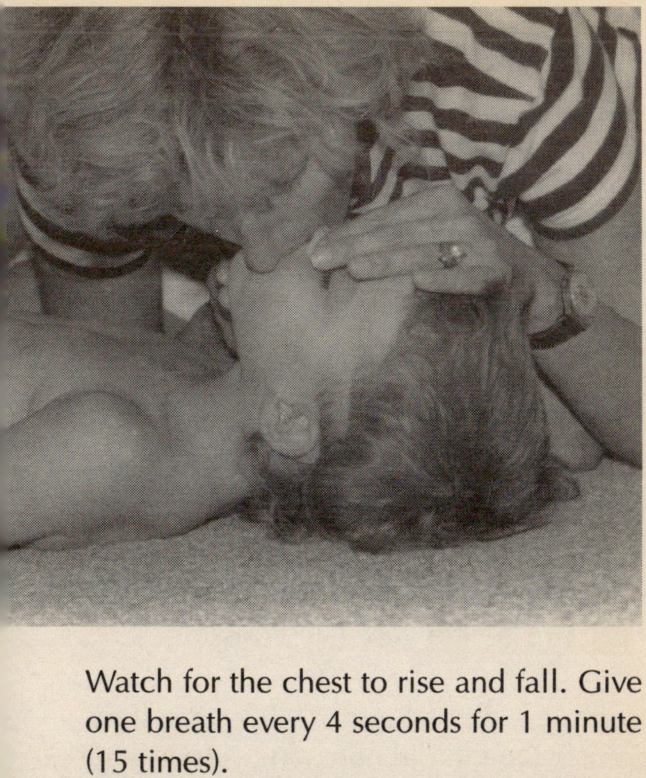

Watch for the chest to rise and fall. Give one breath every 4 seconds for 1 minute (15 times).

To find a heartbeat: Place your head on the child's chest to feel if he is moving or if he is breathing. If he is moving and breathing, stop here.

If no heartbeat, go to STEP 5.

STEP 5

C = COMPRESS

Place the heel of your hand slightly to the left of the breastbone.

Position your shoulders over your hands. Push the heel of your hand down.

Compress chest 5 times. Give one slow breath. Do for 1 minute (10 cycles).

REMEMBER: COUNT OUT LOUD TO KEEP THE RHYTHM.

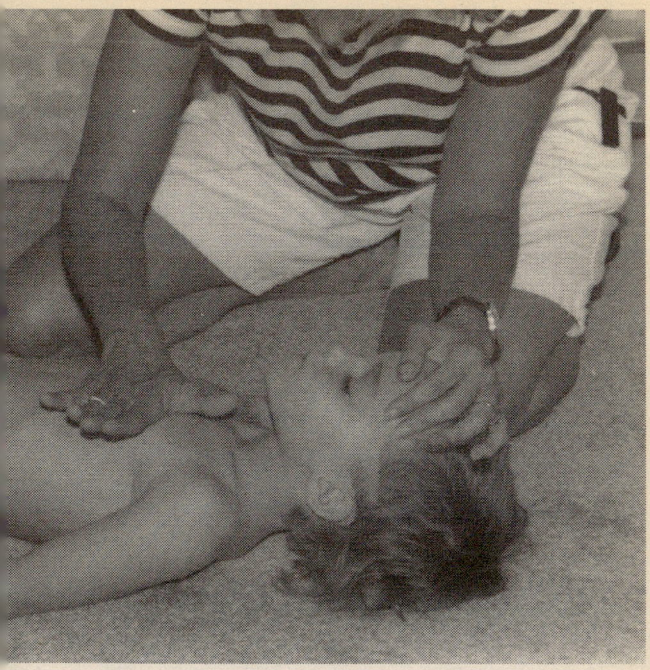

ONE *AND* TWO *AND* THREE *AND* FOUR *AND* FIVE *AND* THEN BREATHE; REPEAT.

The Difference Between Infant and Child CPR

INFANT (Under 1 year)	CHILD (1–8 years)
Observe & Gently Shake Baby	Ask are you okay?
Make Seal over Mouth *and* Nose with Your Mouth	Make Mouth-to-Mouth Seal

COMPRESSIONS:

Draw line between nipples. Place 2 fingers just below make-believe line.	Place heel of your hand slightly to the left of the breastbone.

1 Breath to 5 Compressions:

Quicker in the infant 1-2-3-4-5-Breathe.

Add time between compressions by stating "and" between each number.

1 *and* 2 *and* 3 *and* 4 *and* 5 *and* Breathe.

3

CHOKING

The body has a built-in cough reflex to help dislodge foreign objects that can cause an airway blockage that prevents oxygen-rich air from getting to the lungs. However, sometimes the object is too large to be dislodged by coughing and choking occurs. Sometimes, all measures taken to dislodge the foreign object fail and CPR becomes necessary.

This chapter will help you:

Develop skills to be used when an infant or child chokes.

Develop an understanding of the differences between choking in an infant and in a child.

Review the steps to be taken in applying CPR.

Infant Choking
WHAT DO I DO?

CALL FOR HELP!
DIAL 9·1·1

Determine if the baby is having problems breathing. If the baby is choking and crying, DO NOT INTERFERE. CALL 9-1-1.

STEP 1

(Under 1 year)

If the infant is unable to cry or cough:

Do not try Heimlich Maneuver. Instead:

▶ Hold baby's head down and slap sharply between the baby's shoulder blades. Give 5 back slaps.

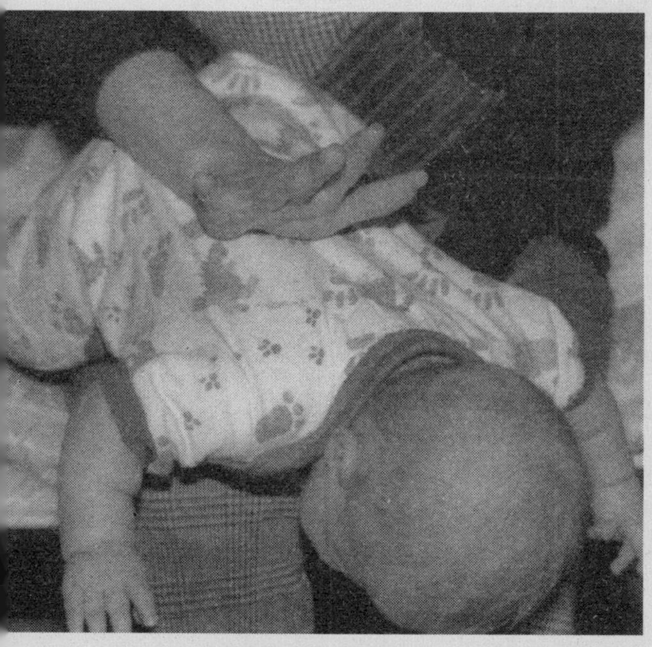

STEP 2

Alternate with 5 chest thrusts

▶ Hold baby on her back with the head lower than the body and push in on the breastbone at the level just below the nipple line.

Repeat these steps until the baby spits out the object or starts breathing.

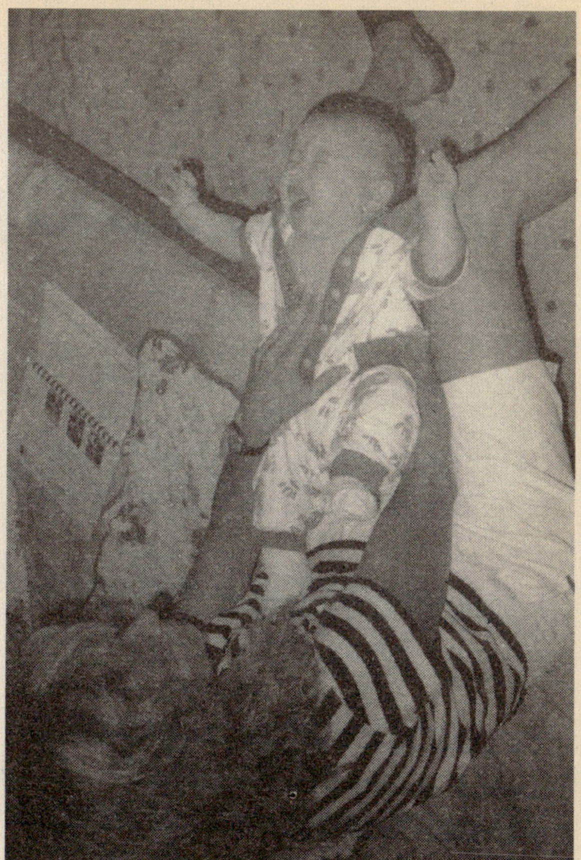

REMEMBER:

NEVER STOP TRYING TO GET THE OBJECT OUT. AS TIME GOES ON, THE BABY WILL BECOME MORE RELAXED AND IT MAY BE EASIER TO DISLODGE THE OBJECT.

KEEP DOING ALTERNATE BACK BLOWS AND CHEST THRUSTS.

IF THE INFANT CAN CRY OR COUGH, DO *NOT* INTERFERE. DO *NOT* TRY TO REMOVE THE OBJECT WITH YOUR FINGER—THIS MAY PUSH THE OBJECT FARTHER DOWN INTO THE THROAT.

IF THE BABY BECOMES LIMP AND STOPS BREATHING, START CPR.

CPR Review

A = AIRWAY

CHECK TO SEE IF THE BABY CAN BREATHE. IF NOT, OPEN AIRWAY.

B = BREATHING

IF THE BABY IS NOT BREATHING, BEGIN RESCUE BREATHING.

GIVE TWO BREATHS:

IF THE CHEST DOES NOT RISE, TRY TO CLEAR THE AIRWAY AGAIN.

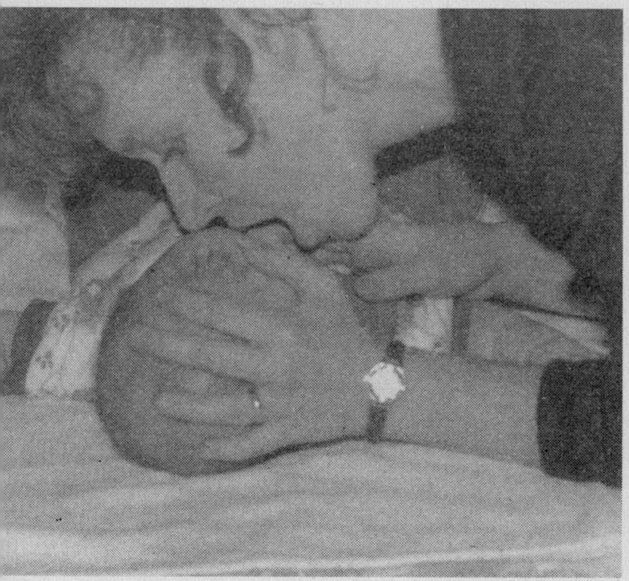

C = COMPRESS

IF THE BABY IS LIMP, NOT BREATHING, AND THERE IS NO HEARTBEAT, BEGIN CHEST COMPRESSIONS.
(See pages 20–24.)

DO NOT FORGET: CALL FOR HELP!

DIAL 9 · 1 · 1

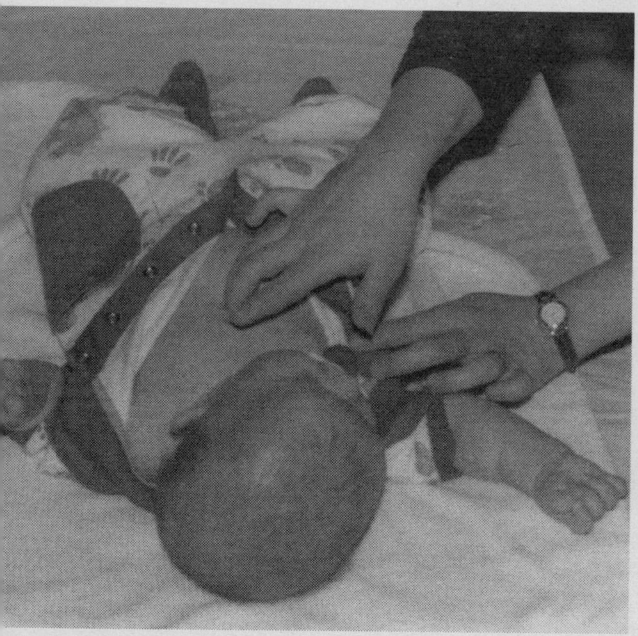

Child Choking
WHAT DO I DO?

CALL FOR HELP!
DIAL 9·1·1

(1 year or older)

Stay with the child and observe him for breathing difficulty. If the child can speak, encourage him to cough. *Do Not Interfere!*

STEP 1

If the child cannot make sounds, you must help.

STEP 2

Begin the Abdominal Thrusts (Heimlich Maneuver).

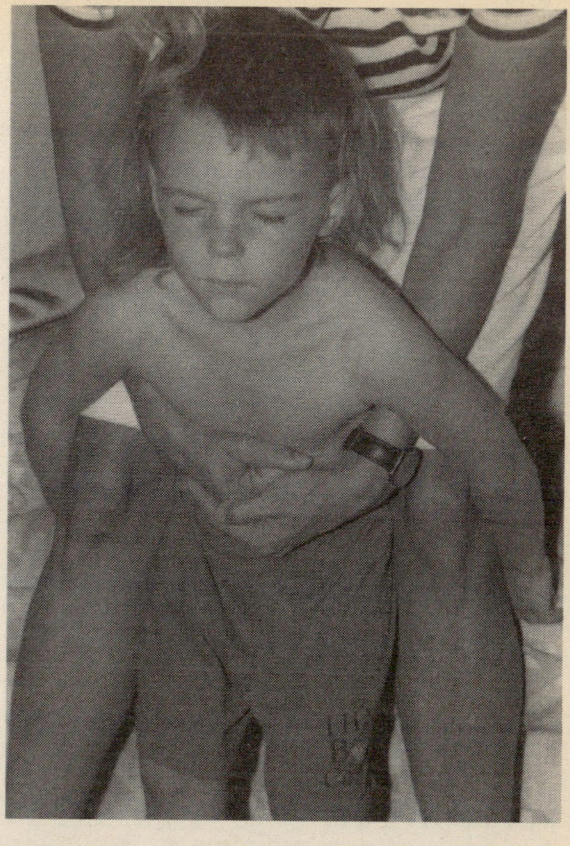

Standing behind the child, wrap your arms around the child's waist. Make a fist with one hand. Put the thumb side of your fist against the child's belly, just above the belly button. Grasp your fist with the other hand. Push your fist into the child's belly with a quick upward movement. Do this 6 to 8 times or until the object is expelled or the child starts to breathe.

BE PERSISTENT! DO NOT STOP!

AS THE CHILD BECOMES MORE DEPRIVED OF OXYGEN, THE MUSCLES WILL BECOME RELAXED AND MEASURES THAT WERE NOT SUCCESSFUL BEFORE MAY NOW WORK.

NEVER GIVE UP!

STEP 3

If the child becomes limp and unable to breathe, begin the steps of CPR.

CPR Review

REMEMBER:

A = AIRWAY

OPEN THE AIRWAY AND DETERMINE IF THE CHILD IS BREATHING.

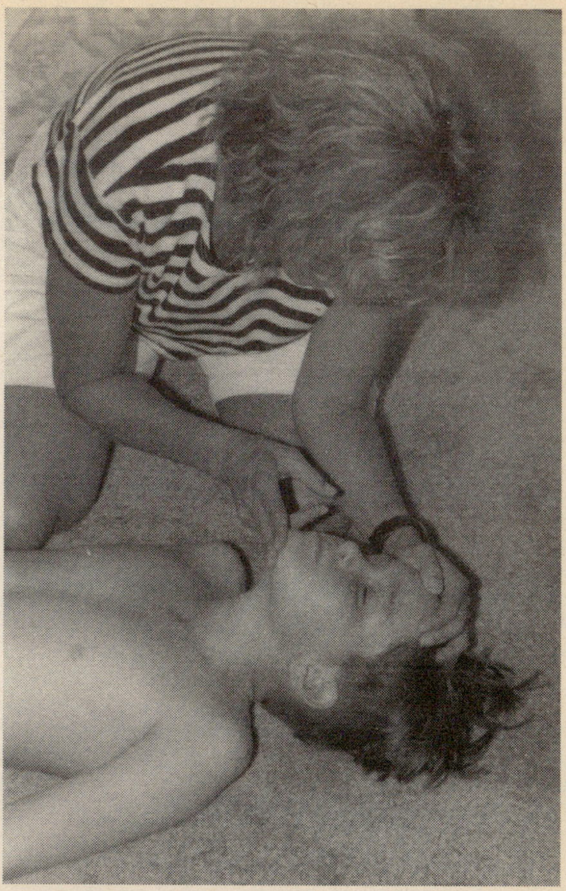

B = BREATHING

DO RESCUE BREATHING, 2 BREATHS (see pages 28–30).

IF CHEST DOES NOT RISE, TRY AGAIN TO CLEAR THE AIRWAY.

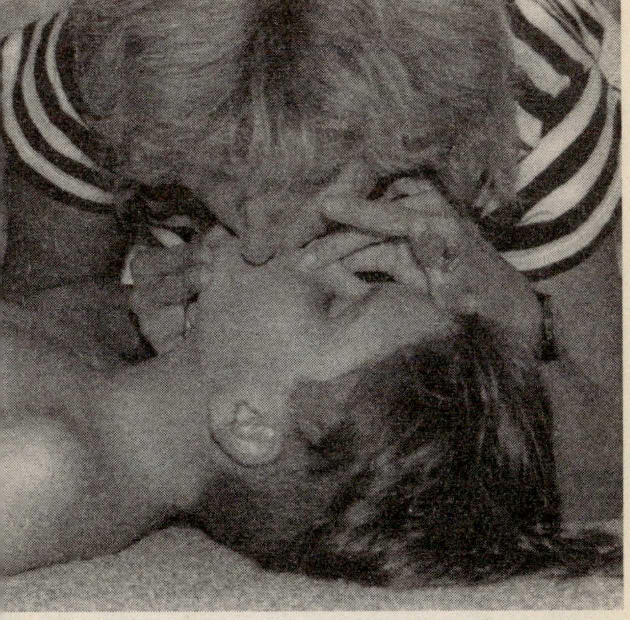

C = COMPRESS

IF THE CHILD'S HEART IS NOT BEATING, BEGIN COMPRESSIONS.

KEEP THE FOLLOWING RHYTHM:

ONE *AND* TWO *AND* THREE *AND* FOUR *AND* FIVE *AND* BREATHE.

DO NOT FORGET TO CALL FOR HELP!

DIAL 9·1·1

STAY CALM!

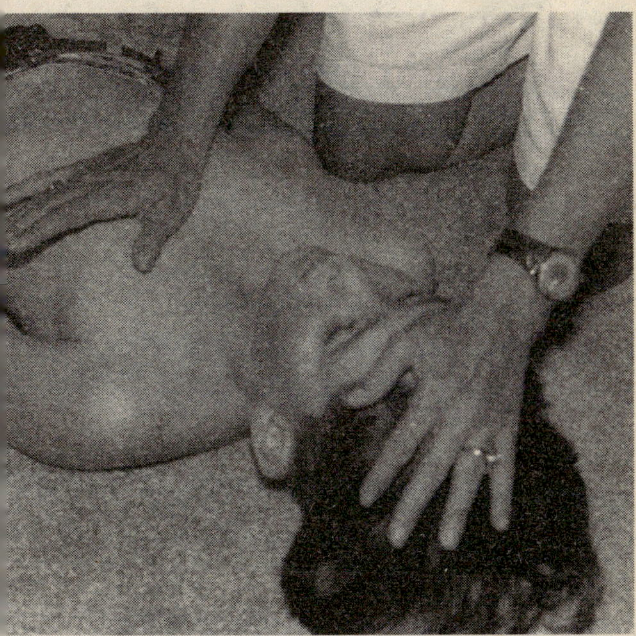

The Difference Between Infant and Child Choking

INFANT	CHILD
BACK BLOWS: 5 back slaps to upper back between shoulder blades	**NO BACK BLOWS**
CHEST THRUSTS: 5 chest thrusts (just below the nipple line) using 2 fingers with baby's head down	**NO CHEST THRUSTS**

INFANT	CHILD
NO ABDOMINAL THRUSTS	**ABDOMINAL THRUSTS (HEIMLICH MANEUVER):** Stand behind child; wrap arms around child's waist. Grasp one fist with your other hand midbelly (above navel). Push inward and upward into belly 6 to 10 times.

4

QUICK REFERENCE

What Parents Have to Say

Some commonly asked questions from parents:

Q. What makes parents take a course in CPR?

A. Most parents take a course in CPR because they have a seriously ill child or infant, are pregnant, or have experienced an infant or child choke or stop breathing.

Q. Do parents have a difficult time learning this skill?

A. In general, parents have the most difficult time learning CPR if their child is ill in the hospital and they are forced to learn the skill quickly. If parents learn in a relaxed manner (either alone or in a group), they do not find learning CPR a very difficult or intimidating skill.

Q. During an emergency, are parents able to perform CPR on their child?

A. The majority of parents questioned feel they know what to do and could perform CPR appropriately. The major concern parents have is their inability to remember the numerous steps and their correct order. The number of times each step is repeated (for example: How many breaths? Where do I take the pulse?) causes confusion to some parents. Most parents called upon to perform CPR did what they instinctively felt was the right thing to do even if the steps of CPR were not performed in an exact order. The majority stated that they were successful in their attempt to resuscitate.

Q. Should parents take a CPR course more than once a year?

A. Parents questioned felt that it would be a good idea to take the course at least twice a year. If this is not possible, all parents should read a manual or see a video on how to perform CPR. They felt that there should be easy reminders around the house to help them recall the steps. An example of this is either a calendar or a poster of the steps of CPR.

Q. What happens if I do CPR incorrectly?

A. Even though you can cause some damage if CPR is done incorrectly, if you do *not* do CPR, your child can die. So, if your child is not breathing, start CPR. Chest compressions can cause a broken rib, but this can be fixed later. You need to keep your child breathing and her heart beating until medical help arrives.

Q. Why are there different compression counts for infants and children?

A. For an infant, the normal heart rate is 100 beats a minute. So count: 1-2-3-4-5-Breathe. For a child, the normal heart rate is about 80 beats per minute. Count 1 *AND* 2 *AND* 3 *AND* 4 *AND* 5 *AND* Breathe.

Q. How hard do I press on my baby's chest?

A. General advice is to push in 1 inch to 1½ inches. This is a difficult concept to understand. Push in on the infant's or child's chest to see the breastbone move downward, then let it come up again.

Q. What happens if I don't know how to find a pulse?

A. This technique is very hard to do on an infant and child. Instead, place your head on the child's or infant's chest and listen carefully for a heartbeat. You can practice this skill at home on your child or infant.

Q. Can I practice CPR at home?

A. Never try to compress your child unless necessary. You can practice this skill on a doll or pillow to see what it feels like. Also, try to give a *doll* mouth-to-mouth resuscitation. *Never practice this on a real child or infant.*

Q. Should I clear the material out of my baby's mouth before I breathe for him?

A. Always clear out whatever is in your baby's or child's mouth first, but only if you can see it. If it isn't visible and you attempt to dislodge it, you could push it even deeper into the trachea.

Q. Does raising my child's arms when he is choking help?

A. It appears that this movement helps to relax your child and opens up the rib cage. The child appears to cough easier and it will give you a minute to compose yourself so that you can move on to chest thrusts or the Heimlich Maneuver.

Q. Does CPR help my baby's heartbeat?

A. Yes, indirectly. The heart is being pumped by you, thereby artificially moving your baby's oxygen-rich blood to his brain.

Q. When should I call 9-1-1?

A. If you know how to breathe for your child, assess him first and then start rescue breathing. Then call 9-1-1. If you are too nervous to begin, call 9-1-1 first and they will help you through the steps of CPR.

Q. Will 9-1-1 know what to do?

A. Remember, not all areas have 9-1-1, so check NOW with your community resources to see what is available. Either the operator, police, or fire department will have people trained in CPR and they will help you.

Q. Can I do the Heimlich Maneuver on my six-month-old?

A. No. Research has shown that the chest thrusts and back slaps are more effective for an infant.

Q. Can I learn CPR from a book?

A. You can learn the basic steps of CPR from this manual; however, I strongly urge you to take a course in CPR or practice on an American Heart Association or American Red Cross dummy to gain comfort. I also urge you to watch a video on infant and child CPR.

Q. When do I stop doing CPR?

A. Never give up! Keep doing CPR until

your child either starts breathing and her heart is beating or medical help arrives. Never stop giving your child a chance!

Emergency Numbers

Fill in the telephone *Emergency Numbers* for your area below.

Place near your telephones for easy access in case of an emergency.

EMERGENCY **9-1-1**

Police ______________________________

Fire ______________________________

Ambulance ______________________________

Doctor ______________________________

Poison ______________________________

Hospital ______________________________

EMERGENCY **9-1-1**

Police ____________________

Fire ____________________

Ambulance ____________________

Doctor ____________________

Poison ____________________

Hospital ____________________

EMERGENCY **9-1-1**

Police ____________________

Fire ____________________

Ambulance ____________________

Doctor ____________________

Poison ____________________

Hospital ____________________

EMERGENCY **9-1-1**

Police ______________________________

Fire ______________________________

Ambulance ______________________________

Doctor ______________________________

Poison ______________________________

Hospital ______________________________

EMERGENCY **9-1-1**

Police ______________________________

Fire ______________________________

Ambulance ______________________________

Doctor ______________________________

Poison ______________________________

Hospital ______________________________

EMERGENCY REFERENCE

Infant CPR

CALL FOR HELP!
DIAL 9·1·1

STEP 1 Gently Shake or Pinch Baby

STEP 2 Open Baby's Airway

A

STEP 3 Check for Breathing:
LOOK
LISTEN
FEEL

STEP 4 Give Air

B

STEP 5 If No Heartbeat, Start Chest Compressions

C

FIVE Compressions then ONE Breath

Count out loud:
ONE · TWO · THREE · FOUR · FIVE · BREATHE.

REPEAT CYCLES
Continue to do this until help arrives or baby has a heartbeat or starts breathing.

DO NOT GIVE UP!

EMERGENCY REFERENCE

Child CPR

CALL FOR HELP!
DIAL 9 · 1 · 1

STEP 1 Gently Shake Child; Ask "Are you okay?"

STEP 2 Open Child's Airway

A

STEP 3 Check for Breathing:
LOOK
LISTEN
FEEL

STEP 4 Give Air

B

STEP 5 If No Heartbeat, Start Chest Compressions

C

FIVE Compressions then ONE Breath.

Count out loud:

ONE *AND* TWO *AND* THREE *AND* FOUR *AND* FIVE *AND* BREATHE.

REPEAT CYCLES
Continue to do this until help arrives or child has a heartbeat and starts to breathe.

DO NOT GIVE UP!